DANIEL TROAST, AUD

Hearing Aid and Hearing Loss Myths Debunked

Separating Fact from Fiction

Copyright © 2024 by Daniel Troast, AuD

All rights reserved. No part of this publication may be reproduced, stored or transmitted in any form or by any means, electronic, mechanical, photocopying, recording, scanning, or otherwise without written permission from the publisher. It is illegal to copy this book, post it to a website, or distribute it by any other means without permission.

Daniel Troast, AuD asserts the moral right to be identified as the author of this work.

Daniel Troast, AuD has no responsibility for the persistence or accuracy of URLs for external or third-party Internet Websites referred to in this publication and does not guarantee that any content on such Websites is, or will remain, accurate or appropriate.

Designations used by companies to distinguish their products are often claimed as trademarks. All brand names and product names used in this book and on its cover are trade names, service marks, trademarks and registered trademarks of their respective owners. The publishers and the book are not associated with any product or vendor mentioned in this book. None of the companies referenced within the book have endorsed the book.

The content of this book is for informational purposes only and is not intended to diagnose, treat, cure, or prevent any condition or disease. You understand that this book is not intended as a substitute for consultation with a licensed practitioner. Please consult with your own physician or healthcare specialist regarding the suggestions and recommendations made in this book. The use of this book implies your acceptance of this disclaimer.

First edition

This book was professionally typeset on Reedsy.
Find out more at reedsy.com

Contents

Introduction	1
Myths about Hearing Loss and the Impacts of Untreated...	2
Myth 1: Only Older Adults Experience Hearing Loss	2
Myth 2: Hearing Loss is Inevitable as You Age	3
Myth 3: Hearing Loss Only Affects Your Ability to Hear	6
Myth 4: Untreated Hearing Loss Isn't a Big Deal	7
Myth 5: Hearing Loss Doesn't Affect Your Quality of Life	8
Myth 6: I Can't Prevent Hearing Loss	10
Myths About Hearing Aids and Hearing Aid Technology	13
Myth 1: Hearing Aids Make You Look Old	13
Myth 2: Hearing Aids Are Only for Severe Hearing Loss	15
Myth 3: Hearing Aids Are Uncomfortable and Inconvenient	17
Myth 4: Hearing Aids Are Just Amplifiers	18
Myth 5: Hearing Aids Can Fully Restore Your Hearing	20
Myth 6: Hearing Aids Are Too Expensive	22
Myth 7: I Can't Wear Hearing Aids Because of My Active Lifestyle	24

Myths Addressing Stigma, Misconceptions, and Objection to... 28
  Myth 1: People Will Treat Me Differently If They Know I Have Hearing Loss 28
  Myth 2: Hearing Aids Will Make My Hearing Worse Over Time 30
  Myth 3: I Can't Afford Hearing Aids, So There's No Point in Getting Tested 33
  Myth 4: I Can Get By Without Hearing Aids 35
  Myth 5: I Don't Want to Admit That I Have Hearing Loss 37
  Myth 6: Hearing Aids Will Make Everything Too Loud 39

Myths of Addressing Hearing Loss 42
  Myth 1: Hearing Aids Will Solve All My Communication Problems 42
  Myth 2: It's Too Late to Address My Hearing Loss 46

Conclusion 49

Resources 50

About the Author 52

Introduction

Welcome to "Hearing Aid and Hearing Loss Myths Debunked: Separating Fact from Fiction." In this book, we will explore and debunk common myths and misconceptions surrounding hearing loss and hearing aids. By separating fact from fiction and using knowledge gained from 20 years of experience, you will be provided a clearer understanding of hearing loss and the benefits of hearing aid use.

Myths about Hearing Loss and the Impacts of Untreated Hearing Loss

Myth 1: Only Older Adults Experience Hearing Loss

Hearing loss is often associated with aging, leading to the misconception that it only affects older adults. However, this is far from the truth. While it is true that hearing loss becomes more prevalent as people age, it can affect individuals of all ages, including children and young adults.

According to the Centers for Disease Control and Prevention (CDC), around 1 to 3 out of every 1,000 children in the United States are born with some degree of hearing loss in one or both ears. Additionally, hearing loss in children can develop later in childhood due to infections, injuries, or exposure to loud noise.

Hearing loss in younger adults can be caused by various factors, including exposure to loud noise, genetics, infections, and medical conditions. Prolonged exposure to loud noise, such as listening to music at high volumes or working in a noisy environment, can damage the delicate structures of the inner ear, leading to hearing loss over time. Infections, such as otitis media (middle ear infection), can cause temporary or permanent hearing loss if left untreated. Additionally, certain medical conditions, such as Ménière's disease or autoimmune disorders, can cause hearing loss in younger adults.

Hearing loss can significantly impact younger adults, affecting their social, emotional, and occupational functioning. In addition to making it difficult to communicate with others, hearing loss can also lead to feelings of isolation, frustration, and depression. In the workplace, hearing loss can affect an individual's ability to perform their job effectively, leading to difficulties with communication, concentration, and productivity.

It is essential for younger adults to be aware of the signs of hearing loss and to seek treatment if they are experiencing symptoms. Early intervention is critical to preventing further damage to the auditory system and minimizing the impact of hearing loss on daily life. Treatment options for hearing loss in younger adults may include hearing aids, assistive listening devices, and cochlear implants, depending on the severity and cause of the hearing loss.

So, our first myth is debunked: hearing loss is not just a problem that affects older adults. It can occur at any age, including in children and younger adults. Raising awareness about the prevalence of hearing loss across all age groups can help ensure that individuals receive the support and treatment they need to live full and healthy lives.

Myth 2: Hearing Loss is Inevitable as You Age

It is a common misconception that hearing loss is an inevitable part of aging. While it is true that hearing loss becomes more prevalent as people age, not everyone will experience significant hearing loss as they get older. Many factors can contribute to hearing loss; some are preventable or manageable with proper care and treatment.

Age-related hearing loss, also known as presbycusis, is the gradual loss of hearing that occurs as people age. It is the most common type of hearing loss and is typically caused by changes to the inner ear due to aging. These changes can include the loss of hair cells in the inner ear, a decrease in blood flow to the inner ear, and changes in the inner ear's structure.

While age is the most significant risk factor for age-related hearing loss, other factors can increase your risk, including exposure to loud noise over time, genetics, smoking, certain medical conditions, such as diabetes and cardiovascular disease, and ototoxic medications, which can damage the inner ear.

While age-related hearing loss may be expected, there are steps you can take to help prevent or minimize it:

1. Protect your ears from loud noise: Limit your exposure to loud noise, and wear ear protection when exposed to loud sounds for extended periods.
2. Get regular hearing screenings: Regular hearing screenings can help detect hearing loss early and allow for early intervention and treatment.
3. Maintain a healthy lifestyle: Eating a balanced diet, exercising regularly, and avoiding smoking can help protect your overall health, including your hearing.
4. Manage chronic health conditions: Certain chronic health conditions, such as diabetes and cardiovascular disease, can increase your risk of hearing loss. Managing these conditions can help protect your hearing.

While age-related hearing loss is not always preventable, there are treatment options available to help manage it:

1. Hearing aids: Hearing aids are small electronic devices that amplify sound and make it easier to hear. They can be programmed to fit your hearing needs and significantly improve your ability to communicate and engage with the world around you.
2. Assistive listening devices: Assistive listening devices, such as amplified telephones and personal listening devices, can help you hear better in specific situations, such as talking on the phone or watching television.
3. Cochlear implants: Cochlear implants are small electronic devices surgically implanted in the inner ear and can provide a sense of sound to people with severe hearing loss.

Another hearing myth debunked is that while age-related hearing loss may be common, it is not inevitable. By taking steps to protect your hearing and seeking treatment if you experience hearing loss, you can help preserve your hearing and continue to enjoy a full and active life as you age.

Myth 3: Hearing Loss Only Affects Your Ability to Hear

Hearing loss is often misunderstood as a condition that only affects an individual's ability to hear sounds. However, hearing loss can have a much broader impact on a person's overall health and well-being, affecting various aspects of their life beyond their hearing ability.

Hearing loss is not just about difficulty hearing sounds; it can affect many aspects of a person's life, including:

1. Communication: Difficulty understanding speech, especially in noisy environments, can lead to conversation misunderstandings and frustration.
2. Social Isolation: Hearing loss can make it challenging to participate in social activities, leading to feelings of loneliness and isolation.
3. Emotional Well-being: Untreated hearing loss has been linked to an increased risk of depression, anxiety, and other mental health issues.
4. Cognitive Function: There is growing evidence to suggest that untreated hearing loss may be associated with cognitive decline and an increased risk of dementia. Recent research has highlighted a strong connection between untreated hearing loss and cognitive decline. A study by Johns Hopkins Medicine found that older adults with untreated hearing loss were more likely to experience cognitive decline and develop dementia than those without hearing loss. The exact mechanism behind this connection is still not fully understood, but it is believed that the brain's increased effort to process sounds may contribute

to cognitive decline over time.
5. Physical Health: Hearing loss has been linked to an increased risk of falls, accidents, and other physical health problems.

Given the far-reaching impact of hearing loss, it is essential to address it as soon as possible. Fortunately, many effective treatment options are available for hearing loss, including hearing aids and assistive listening devices.

So clearly, this myth is debunked because hearing loss is not just about difficulty hearing sounds; it can significantly impact many aspects of a person's life, including communication, social interaction, emotional well-being, cognitive function, and physical health. By addressing hearing loss early and seeking treatment, individuals can improve their quality of life and reduce their risk of associated health problems.

Myth 4: Untreated Hearing Loss Isn't a Big Deal

Untreated hearing loss is a common but often overlooked health issue. Many people believe hearing loss is simply a part of getting older and is not a serious problem. However, the reality is that untreated hearing loss can have a significant impact on a person's overall health and well-being, affecting various aspects of their life.

While hearing loss may seem like a minor inconvenience, it can have far-reaching consequences if left untreated. Some of the potential consequences of untreated hearing loss, which were covered in the previous myth, include communication difficulties, social isolation, cognitive decline, and negative impact on emotional well-being.

Additionally, untreated hearing loss can result in a reduced quality of life. It can affect their relationships, ability to work and participate in social activities, and overall well-being.

Untreated hearing loss is not a minor issue; it can significantly impact a person's health and well-being. By seeking treatment for their hearing loss, individuals can improve their quality of life, reduce their risk of associated health problems, and actively engage in the world around them. It is essential to raise awareness about the importance of early intervention and to encourage people to seek help if they are experiencing symptoms of hearing loss.

Myth 5: Hearing Loss Doesn't Affect Your Quality of Life

Hearing loss is often perceived as a minor inconvenience that does not significantly impact a person's quality of life. However, the reality is that hearing loss can have a profound effect on various aspects of daily life, including communication, social interactions, emotional well-being, and overall health.

One of the most significant ways that hearing loss affects quality of life is through communication difficulties. Hearing loss can make it challenging to understand speech, especially in noisy environments or when multiple people are talking simultaneously. This can lead to misunderstandings, frustration, and a sense of isolation.

People with hearing loss may struggle to follow conversations in social settings, leading them to withdraw from social activities and avoid gatherings altogether. Over time, this can lead to feelings of loneliness, depression, and anxiety.

Untreated hearing loss can also strain relationships with family members, friends, and colleagues. Communication breakdowns due to hearing loss can lead to misunderstandings and frustration, putting a strain on personal and professional relationships.

People with untreated hearing loss may find it challenging to communicate with their loved ones, leading to feelings of isolation and disconnection. This can further exacerbate feelings of loneliness and depression, ultimately affecting their overall quality of life.

The emotional toll of hearing loss should not be underestimated. People with untreated hearing loss may experience a range of emotions, including frustration, embarrassment, and anxiety. They may feel embarrassed about their condition and may avoid social situations out of fear of not being able to hear or understand what is being said.

Over time, the stress and anxiety caused by untreated hearing loss can take a toll on a person's emotional well-being, leading to depression and other mental health issues. Studies have shown that untreated hearing loss is associated with an increased risk of depression, anxiety, and other psychological problems.

The consequences of untreated hearing loss underscore the importance of seeking treatment as soon as possible. Fortunately, many effective treatment options are available for hearing loss, including hearing aids.

Another myth debunked as we can see that hearing loss can have a significant impact on a person's quality of life, affecting their communication, social interactions, and emotional well-being. It is essential to recognize the importance of seeking hearing loss treatment and taking steps to address it as soon as possible. By seeking treatment for their hearing loss, individuals can improve their quality of life, reduce their risk of associated health problems, and actively engage in the world around them.

Myth 6: I Can't Prevent Hearing Loss

While it is true that some types of hearing loss are inevitable, many cases of hearing loss can be prevented by taking simple steps to protect your ears and maintain good hearing health. Understanding the common causes of hearing loss and taking proactive measures to protect your hearing can significantly reduce your risk of experiencing hearing loss later in life.

Hearing loss can be caused by a variety of factors, including:

1. Exposure to loud noise: Prolonged exposure to loud noise is one of the leading causes of hearing loss. This can include exposure to loud music, construction noise, power tools, and other sources of loud noise.
2. Age-related changes: As people age, they may experience changes to the inner ear that can lead to hearing loss. While age-related hearing loss is common, it is not inevitable, and there are steps you can take to reduce your risk.
3. Genetics: Some types of hearing loss are hereditary and may run in families. If you have a family history of hearing loss, you may be at a higher risk of experiencing hearing loss yourself. So while we may be aware of a family history of heart disease and taking precautions against that, we need also to be mindful of a family history of hearing loss so that we can take any necessary precautions there as well.

4. Medical conditions: Certain conditions, such as diabetes, cardiovascular disease, and infections, can increase your risk of hearing loss.
5. Ototoxic medications: Some medications can damage the delicate structures of the inner ear and lead to hearing loss. These are known as ototoxic medications, including some antibiotics, chemotherapy drugs, and pain relievers. So, if you have any concerns, address them with your prescribing doctor.

While you may not be able to prevent all cases of hearing loss, there are many steps you can take to protect your hearing and reduce your risk of experiencing hearing loss later in life:

1. Protect your ears from loud noise: Limit your exposure to loud noise, and wear ear protection when exposed to loud sounds for extended periods. This can include wearing earplugs or earmuffs when attending concerts, sporting events, or other loud activities.
2. Turn down the volume: When listening to music or watching television, keep the volume at a safe level. Generally, if you have to raise your voice to be heard over the sound, the volume is too loud.
3. Take breaks from loud noise: If you are exposed to loud noise for an extended period, take breaks to rest your ears. This can help prevent damage to the delicate structures of the inner ear.
4. Get regular hearing screenings: Regular hearing screenings can help detect hearing loss early and allow for early intervention and treatment. Be sure to schedule regular check-ups with your doctor and ask for a hearing screening

if you have concerns about your hearing.
5. Maintain a healthy lifestyle: Eating a balanced diet, exercising regularly, and avoiding smoking can help protect your overall health, including your hearing.

While some types of hearing loss are inevitable, the myth is debunked because many cases can be prevented by taking simple steps to protect your ears and maintain good hearing health. Understanding the common causes of hearing loss and taking proactive measures to protect your hearing can significantly reduce your risk of experiencing hearing loss later in life. It is essential to recognize the importance of hearing health and to take steps to protect your hearing at every age.

Myths About Hearing Aids and Hearing Aid Technology

Myth 1: Hearing Aids Make You Look Old

One of the most persistent myths surrounding hearing aids is that wearing them will make you look old. This misconception often leads people to delay seeking treatment for their hearing loss out of fear of being perceived as old or less capable. The perception that hearing aids make you look old is rooted in outdated stereotypes and stigmas surrounding hearing loss. In the past, hearing aids were large, bulky devices that were highly visible when worn. However, technological advances have led to the development of smaller, more discreet hearing aids that are barely noticeable. In fact, with how discreet hearing aids are now, it generally makes you look older and less capable to be consistently misunderstanding and asking for things to be repeated.

In addition to being more discreet, modern hearing aids offer a range of features and benefits that make them more comfortable and convenient to wear:

1. Wireless connectivity: Many modern hearing aids are

equipped with wireless connectivity, allowing them to connect directly to smartphones, televisions, and other electronic devices.
2. Noise reduction technology: Advanced noise reduction technology helps to manage background noise, making it easier to hear speech in noisy environments.
3. Automatic adjustment: Some hearing aids are equipped with automatic adjustment features that adapt to different listening environments, ensuring optimal sound quality at all times.
4. Rechargeable batteries: Many modern hearing aids come with rechargeable batteries, eliminating the need for disposable batteries and making them more convenient.

It is important to challenge the misconception that wearing hearing aids makes you look old and to empower individuals to seek treatment for their hearing loss. Hearing loss is a common condition that can affect people of all ages, and wearing hearing aids should not be a source of shame or embarrassment. Thankfully, this myth is debunked as attitudes toward hearing loss are slowly changing, thanks in part to increased awareness and advocacy efforts and technology's role in our lives as it is more common for people to wear technology on their ears, whether it be a hearing aid or Bluetooth earbud.

Myth 2: Hearing Aids Are Only for Severe Hearing Loss

One of the most common misconceptions about hearing aids is that they are only suitable for people with severe hearing loss. However, the reality is that hearing aids come in various styles and models, each designed to address different degrees of hearing loss. Whether you have mild, moderate, or severe hearing loss, a hearing aid can help you hear better and improve your quality of life.

Before we delve into the various types of hearing aids, it's essential to understand the different degrees of hearing loss:

1. Mild Hearing Loss: People with mild hearing loss may have difficulty hearing soft or distant sounds, such as whispers or quiet conversations.
2. Moderate Hearing Loss: People with moderate hearing loss may have difficulty hearing normal conversational speech, especially in noisy environments.
3. Severe Hearing Loss: People with severe hearing loss may only be able to hear very loud sounds or not hear at all without hearing aids.

There are several types of hearing aids available, each designed to address different degrees of hearing loss and individual preferences. Some of the most common types of hearing aids include:

1. Behind-the-Ear (BTE) or Receiver-in-the-Ear (RIC) Hearing Aids: These hearing aids are the most common type of hearing aid and are suitable for all degrees of hearing loss. They consist of a small plastic case that sits behind the ear and is

connected to an earpiece that fits inside the ear canal.

3. In-the-Canal (ITC) Hearing Aids: ITC hearing aids fit partially inside the ear canal and partially in the bowl of the outer ear. They are suitable for mild to moderate hearing loss.

4. Completely-in-the-Canal (CIC) Hearing Aids: CIC hearing aids are the smallest type of hearing aid available. They are positioned completely inside the ear canal and are appropriate for mild to moderate hearing loss.

While hearing aids are often associated with severe hearing loss, they can also benefit people with mild to moderate hearing loss. Some of the benefits of wearing hearing aids for mild to moderate hearing loss include:

1. Improved Communication: Hearing aids can help people with mild to moderate hearing loss hear and understand speech more distinctly, making communication with others easier.
2. Better Quality of Life: Hearing aids can improve a person's quality of life by allowing them to participate more fully in social activities and engage with the world around them.
3. Slower Rate of Hearing Loss Progression: Untreated hearing loss can further damage the auditory system over time. Wearing hearing aids can help reduce further hearing loss and preserve the remaining hearing ability.
4. Increased Safety: Hearing aids can help people with mild to moderate hearing loss hear important sounds, such as alarms, doorbells, and traffic signals, reducing their risk of accidents and injuries.

This myth is easily debunked; hearing aids are not just for people with severe hearing loss; they can also benefit people with mild to moderate hearing loss. Whether you have mild, moderate, or severe hearing loss, a hearing aid can help you hear better and improve your quality of life. If you are experiencing difficulty hearing, don't hesitate to talk to your audiologist about whether hearing aids may suit you.

Myth 3: Hearing Aids Are Uncomfortable and Inconvenient

Another common misconception about hearing aids is that they are uncomfortable and inconvenient. While it is true that some people may experience initial discomfort when first wearing hearing aids, modern advancements in hearing aid technology have made them more comfortable and convenient to use than ever before.

Today's hearing aids are smaller, more discreet, and more technologically advanced than ever. They come in various styles and models, each designed to address different degrees of hearing loss and individual preferences. Some of the features of modern hearing aids include:

1. Comfortable fit: Modern hearing aids are custom-made or measured to fit comfortably in your ear, reducing the risk of discomfort or irritation. They are designed to be worn all day without causing discomfort.
2. Advanced technology: Modern hearing aids have advanced digital technology that enhances sound quality and reduces background noise. They can be programmed to fit your hearing needs and automatically adjust to different listening environments.

3. Wireless connectivity: Many modern hearing aids are equipped with wireless connectivity, allowing them to connect directly to smartphones, televisions, and other electronic devices. This will enable you to stream audio directly to your hearing aids, making it easier to hear phone calls, music, and other audio content.

So, we can add to the list of debunked myths that hearing aids are uncomfortable and d inconvenient. Modern advancements in hearing aid technology have made them smaller, more discreet, and more comfortable than ever before. If you are experiencing difficulty hearing, don't let misconceptions about hearing aids hold you back.

Myth 4: Hearing Aids Are Just Amplifiers

Another frequent misconception about hearing aids is that they are simply amplifiers that make sounds louder. While it is true that hearing aids do amplify sounds, modern hearing aids are much more sophisticated than simple amplifiers. They are equipped with advanced digital technology that enhances sound quality, reduces background noise, and provides a more natural listening experience.

To understand why the idea that hearing aids are just amplifiers is a myth, it's essential to understand how hearing aids work. While older analog hearing aids primarily amplify sounds, modern digital hearing aids work differently. Here's how they work:

1. Sound reception: The microphone on the hearing aid picks

up sounds from the environment.
2. Sound processing: The hearing aid processes the sounds using advanced digital signal processing algorithms. These algorithms analyze the sounds and adjust them based on the individual's hearing loss, listening environment, and preferences.
3. Sound amplification: The processed sounds are then amplified to make them audible to the wearer. However, modern hearing aids do not simply make sounds louder; they amplify specific frequencies based on the individual's hearing loss and listening needs.
4. Sound delivery: The amplified sounds are delivered to the ear through a speaker or earpiece, allowing the wearer to hear more clearly.

Modern hearing aids are equipped with a range of advanced features and technologies that go beyond simple amplification. Some of these features include:

1. Directional microphones: Many modern hearing aids have directional microphones that focus on speech while reducing background noise. This helps improve speech understanding in noisy environments.
2. Noise reduction: Advanced noise reduction algorithms help reduce background noise, making it easier to hear speech in challenging listening situations.
3. Feedback cancellation: Feedback cancellation technology helps prevent whistling and feedback noises that can occur with older hearing aids.

The advanced features and technologies in modern hearing aids offer a range of benefits for people with hearing loss that are better than amplifiers. These benefits include improved speech understanding, reduced background noise, improved sound quality, and increased comfort and convenience.

While it is true that hearing aids amplify sounds, this myth is debunked because they are much more than simple amplifiers. Modern hearing aids have advanced digital technology that enhances sound quality, reduces background noise, and provides a more natural listening experience. They are designed with the specific needs of hearing-loss individuals in mind and improve their quality of life.

Myth 5: Hearing Aids Can Fully Restore Your Hearing

While hearing aids are highly effective at improving hearing and enhancing communication for people with hearing loss, they cannot fully restore normal hearing. Despite significant advancements in hearing aid technology, there are limitations to what hearing aids can achieve. Understanding these limitations is essential for managing expectations and making informed decisions about hearing healthcare.

To understand why the idea that hearing aids can fully restore your hearing is a myth, it's essential to understand the nature of hearing loss. Hearing loss can be caused by damage to the outer ear, middle ear, inner ear, or auditory nerve, varying in severity from mild to profound.

While hearing aids can help people with mild to severe hearing loss hear better and improve their quality of life, they cannot fully restore normal hearing. Here's why:

MYTHS ABOUT HEARING AIDS AND HEARING AID TECHNOLOGY

1. Amplification vs. Restoration: Hearing aids amplify sounds to make them audible to the wearer. While they can make sounds louder and clearer, they cannot restore the underlying damage to the auditory system that caused the hearing loss in the first place.
2. Complexity of Hearing: The process of hearing is complex and involves the transmission of sound waves through the outer ear, middle ear, inner ear, and auditory nerve to the brain. Hearing aids can help compensate for damage to the inner ear and auditory nerve, but they cannot repair or restore this damage.
3. Degree of Hearing Loss: The effectiveness of hearing aids depends on the degree and type of hearing loss. While hearing aids can provide significant benefits for people with mild to moderate hearing loss, their effectiveness may be limited for people with severe to profound hearing loss.

While hearing aids cannot fully restore normal hearing, they can provide significant benefits for people with hearing loss, including improved communication and social interaction, better quality of life and emotional well-being, increased safety and independence, prevention of further hearing loss, and enhanced cognitive function and brain health.

So, while there are many benefits to wearing hearing aids, the idea that hearing aids can return your hearing ability to what it once was is a myth. While hearing aids are highly effective at improving hearing and enhancing communication for people with hearing loss, they cannot fully restore normal hearing.

Myth 6: Hearing Aids Are Too Expensive

One myth that stops many people from pursuing correction for their hearing loss is the idea hearing aids are too expensive for the average person to afford. While it's true that hearing aids can be a significant investment, many options are available at various price points to fit different budgets. Financial assistance programs, insurance coverage, and other resources are available to help make hearing aids more affordable for those who need them.

The cost of hearing aids can vary widely depending on several factors, including:

1. Technology level: Hearing aids are available in a variety technology levels, ranging from basic to premium. Premium hearing aids typically come with more advanced features and technologies, which can increase their cost.
2. Additional features: Some hearing aids come with additional features, such as rechargeable batteries, remote controls, and smartphone compatibility, which can increase their cost.
3. Professional fees: The cost of hearing aids often includes the services of an audiologist or hearing aid specialist, who will conduct a hearing evaluation, recommend the appropriate hearing aids, and provide fitting and follow-up care to ensure success with the hearing aid you choose.

Despite the availability of affordable options, many people still perceive hearing aids as being too expensive. Several factors contribute to this perception, including:

1. Lack of insurance coverage: Insurance plans do not always cover the cost of hearing aids, leaving people to pay out of pocket. However, many insurance plans now offer some coverage for hearing aids.
2. Limited financial resources: For people on fixed incomes or with limited financial resources, the cost of hearing aids can be prohibitive, even if they are technically affordable.
3. Misconceptions about hearing aids: Many people are unaware of the range of options available and assume that they are all expensive. Additionally, some people may not realize that financial assistance programs and other resources are available to help make hearing aids more affordable.

While the cost of hearing aids can be a significant barrier for many people, there are several options available to help make them more affordable:

1. Insurance coverage: As just mentioned, many insurance plans now offer some coverage for hearing aids.
2. Financial assistance programs: Several financial assistance programs are available to help make hearing aids more affordable for those who need them. These programs may offer discounted or free hearing aids to qualifying individuals.
3. Flexible spending accounts (FSAs) and health savings accounts (HSAs): Many employers offer FSAs and HSAs, which allow you to set aside pre-tax dollars to pay for medical expenses, including hearing aids.
4. Veterans benefits: Veterans may be eligible for hearing aids through the Department of Veterans Affairs (VA)

healthcare system.

So, the idea that hearing aids are too expensive is a myth that has been debunked. While hearing aids can be a significant investment, many options are available at various prices to fit different budgets. Financial assistance programs, insurance coverage, and other resources are available to help make hearing aids more affordable for those who need them.

Myth 7: I Can't Wear Hearing Aids Because of My Active Lifestyle

Another misperception about hearing aids is that they are unsuitable for people with active lifestyles. Some believe hearing aids will be uncomfortable, easily damaged, or inconvenient during physical activities. However, modern hearing aids are designed to be durable, comfortable, and versatile, making them suitable for people with even the most active lifestyles.

Before we explore why this myth is untrue, it's essential to understand the concerns that some people have about wearing hearing aids while being active:

1. Discomfort: Some individuals worry that hearing aids will be uncomfortable to wear during physical activities, such as exercise or sports.
2. Durability: Others are concerned that hearing aids will be easily damaged by sweat, moisture, or impact during physical activities.
3. Inconvenience: Some worry that hearing aids will be inconvenient to wear during physical activities, such as

swimming or playing sports.

Contrary to popular belief, the design of modern hearing aids is suitable for people with even the most active lifestyles. Here's why:

1. Durability: Modern hearing aids are built to withstand the rigors of daily life, including physical activities. Many hearing aids are water-resistant or even waterproof, making them suitable for activities such as swimming and water sports. Additionally, many hearing aids come with protective coatings or nano-coatings that repel moisture and sweat, helping to prevent damage and extending the life of the hearing aid.
2. Comfort: Comfort is a top priority when designing hearing aids for active individuals. Many modern hearing aids are small, lightweight, and designed to fit comfortably in the ear. They are custom-made to fit the contours of your ear, reducing the risk of discomfort or irritation during physical activities. Additionally, many hearing aids come in different sizes and styles, including ear tips and domes, allowing you to find the perfect fit for your ears.
3. Versatility: Modern hearing aids are incredibly versatile, with features and technologies that make them suitable for a wide range of activities. Many hearing aids come with advanced noise reduction algorithms that can help manage background noise, making it easier to hear speech in noisy environments such as gyms or sports fields. Additionally, many hearing aids have directional microphones that can focus on speech while reducing background noise, further improving speech understanding during physical

activities.

There are many benefits to wearing hearing aids during physical activities, including:

- Improved safety: Hearing essential sounds, such as approaching vehicles or emergency sirens, can help keep you safe during physical activities.

- Enhanced communication: Hearing aids can help you communicate more effectively with coaches, teammates, and other participants during sports and other physical activities.

- Increased enjoyment: Being able to hear and engage fully in physical activities can make them more enjoyable and rewarding.

- Better overall health: Regular physical activity is essential for maintaining good health and well-being. Hearing and participating fully in physical activities can help improve your physical fitness and quality of life.

Here are some tips for wearing hearing aids during physical activities:

1. Choose the right hearing aids: Look for hearing aids specifically designed for active lifestyles, with features such as water resistance, moisture resistance, and durability.
2. Secure your hearing aids: Use retention clips, ear hooks, or other accessories to secure them during physical activities and prevent them from falling out.
3. Protect your hearing aids: Consider using a protective case or pouch to store them when not in use, especially during activities where they may be exposed to moisture or impact.

Modern technology easily allows us to debunk the idea that

you can't wear hearing aids because you're too active. Modern hearing aids are designed to be durable, comfortable, and versatile, making them suitable for people with even the most active lifestyles. By choosing the right hearing aids and taking proper precautions, you can enjoy the benefits of improved hearing during physical activities without sacrificing comfort or convenience.

Myths Addressing Stigma, Misconceptions, and Objection to Correction

Myth 1: People Will Treat Me Differently If They Know I Have Hearing Loss

A common concern people with hearing loss have is that others will treat them differently if they know about their hearing impairment. This fear can result in feelings of isolation, embarrassment, and reluctance to seek help for hearing loss. However, in reality, most people are understanding and accommodating once they are aware of someone's hearing loss, and being open about your hearing impairment can lead to better communication and stronger relationships.

Before we dispel this myth, let's understand the concerns that people with hearing loss may have about disclosing their condition:

1. Fear of stigma: Some people worry that others will judge or treat them differently if they know about their hearing loss, leading to embarrassment or shame.

2. Communication barriers: Others may worry that their hearing loss will make it difficult to communicate with others, leading to awkward or uncomfortable interactions.
3. Impact on relationships: Some people may worry that hearing loss will strain their relationships with friends, family, and coworkers, leading to isolation and loneliness.

Now that we understand why an individual with hearing loss doesn't want to disclose their hearing difficulty, we can break down why they shouldn't be concerned, and here's why:

1. Increased understanding: People aware of your hearing loss are more likely to make accommodations to ensure effective communication. This may include speaking more clearly, facing you when they speak, and speaking louder if necessary.
2. Improved communication: Being open about your hearing loss allows you to communicate more effectively with others. It allows you to explain your communication needs and preferences, making it easier for others to understand and accommodate your hearing impairment.
3. Strengthened relationships: Being open about hearing loss can help strengthen relationships with friends, family, and coworkers. It allows others to understand your needs and challenges better, fostering empathy, understanding, and support.

Here are some tips for disclosing your hearing loss to others:

1. Choose the right time and place: Pick a quiet, private setting where you can have a conversation without dis-

tractions.
2. Be direct and honest: Be open and honest about your hearing loss, and explain how it affects your communication and daily life.
3. Educate others: Take the opportunity to educate others about hearing loss and how they can help you communicate more effectively.

The idea that people will treat you differently if they know you have hearing loss is a myth. Most people are understanding and accommodating when they learn that someone has hearing loss, and being open about your hearing impairment can lead to better communication and stronger relationships. Don't let fear of stigma or judgment hold you back from disclosing your hearing loss to others. Being open and honest about your hearing impairment can improve communication, reduce stress and anxiety, and strengthen relationships.

Myth 2: Hearing Aids Will Make My Hearing Worse Over Time

One of the most persistent myths surrounding hearing aids is the belief that wearing them will worsen your hearing over time. This misconception can lead to reluctance to seek help for hearing loss and can prevent people from experiencing the many benefits that hearing aids offer. However, no evidence supports the idea that wearing hearing aids will make your hearing worse over time. The opposite is true: wearing hearing aids can help slow further deterioration of your hearing and improve your overall hearing health.

Before we debunk this myth, let's explore the concerns that some people have about wearing hearing aids:

1. Dependency: Some people worry that wearing hearing aids will make them dependent on amplification and cause their natural hearing to deteriorate over time.
2. Adaptation: Others worry that wearing hearing aids will cause their ears to become accustomed to amplified sound, making it more difficult to hear without them.
3. Damage: Some people worry that wearing hearing aids will damage their ears or cause further hearing deterioration over time.

So now that we understand the why behind this myth, we can easily break down why the evidence doesn't support the claim. Hearing aids can help prevent further hearing deterioration and improve your hearing health. Here's why:

1. Preventing Auditory Deprivation

One of the main reasons why wearing hearing aids can actually help slow further deterioration of your hearing is because it prevents auditory deprivation. Auditory deprivation occurs when the auditory system is deprived of stimulation due to untreated hearing loss. Over time, this lack of stimulation can further deteriorate your hearing. Wearing hearing aids helps counteract the impact of auditory deprivation.

2. Auditory Stimulation

Wearing hearing aids provides your auditory system with the stimulation it needs to remain active and healthy. By amplifying sounds and making them audible, hearing aids help keep your auditory system engaged and active, preventing auditory deprivation and deterioration of your hearing over time.

3. Auditory Plasticity

The auditory system is incredibly adaptable, and wearing hearing aids can help facilitate auditory plasticity. Auditory plasticity refers to the brain's ability to adapt and reorganize in response to changes in auditory input. By providing your auditory system with the stimulation it needs, hearing aids can help facilitate auditory plasticity and improve your overall hearing health.

4. Regular Auditory Stimulation

Wearing hearing aids ensures that your auditory system receives regular stimulation, essential for maintaining good hearing health. By amplifying sounds and making them audible, hearing aids help keep your auditory system active and engaged, preventing auditory deprivation and deterioration of your hearing over time.

The idea that hearing aids will make your hearing worse over time is a myth debunked. There is no evidence to support this belief, and in fact, wearing hearing aids can help reduce further deterioration of your hearing and improve your overall hearing health.

Myth 3: I Can't Afford Hearing Aids, So There's No Point in Getting Tested

While it's true that hearing aids can be a significant investment, there are many reasons why getting tested for hearing loss is still important, even if you can't afford hearing aids. Identifying hearing loss early can lead to better outcomes and positively impact your overall quality of life, regardless of whether you choose to pursue hearing aids or other treatment options.

Before we debunk this myth, let's explore the concerns that some people have about getting tested for hearing loss:

1. Cost: Many people worry that getting tested for hearing loss will be expensive and that they won't be able to afford treatment, such as hearing aids.
2. Time: Some people worry that getting tested for hearing loss will take too much time and effort, especially if they don't think they can afford treatment.
3. Stigma: Others worry that getting tested for hearing loss will make their condition more real or that they will be stigmatized if they are diagnosed with hearing loss.

Even though many still believe the contrary, there are many reasons why getting tested for hearing loss is still important, even if you can't afford hearing aids. Identifying hearing loss early can lead to better outcomes and improve your overall quality of life, regardless of whether you choose to pursue hearing aids or other treatment options. Here's why:

1. Early Detection

Getting tested for hearing loss allows you to identify the problem early and take steps to address it before it worsens.

Early detection of hearing loss can lead to better outcomes and may even prevent further hearing deterioration over time.

2. Improved Communication

Even if you can't afford hearing aids, knowing that you have hearing loss allows you to take steps to improve communication and make adjustments in your daily life. For example, you can:

- Ask people to speak more clearly and face you when they speak.
- Avoid noisy environments whenever possible.
- Use visual cues like lip reading and facial expressions to help understand speech.

3. Access to Resources and Support

Getting tested for hearing loss allows you to access resources and support that can help you manage your condition and improve your quality of life. For example, you may be eligible for financial assistance programs, support groups, and other resources to help you cope with hearing loss and improve your communication skills.

4. Identifying Underlying Health Issues

In some cases, hearing loss may be a symptom of an underlying health issue, such as an ear infection or a problem with the auditory nerve. Getting tested for hearing loss allows you to identify these underlying health issues and take steps to address them before they worsen.

The notion that there's no reason to get tested for hearing loss if you can't afford hearing aids is a debunked myth. Identifying hearing loss early can lead to better outcomes and improve your overall quality of life, regardless of whether you choose to pursue hearing aids or other treatment options.

Myth 4: I Can Get By Without Hearing Aids

Some people say they can "get by" without using hearing aids. Many people think their hearing loss isn't severe enough to warrant hearing aids, or they can manage it with strategies like lip reading and turning up the volume on electronic devices. However, untreated hearing loss can lead to numerous negative consequences that significantly affect one's quality of life. Here's why getting by without hearing aids isn't a viable solution for most people with hearing loss.

Hearing loss isn't just an inconvenience; it's a condition that can affect various aspects of your life:

1. Communication: The most immediate impact of hearing loss is on your ability to communicate effectively. Difficulty hearing can lead to frequent misunderstandings and frustrations in conversations, making it challenging to maintain relationships.
2. Cognitive Decline: Studies have shown a link between untreated hearing loss and cognitive decline, including an increased risk of dementia. The brain has to work harder to process sounds, which can reduce cognitive resources available for other tasks.
3. Social Isolation: Difficulty hearing can make social interactions exhausting and less enjoyable, leading many to withdraw from social activities. This isolation can result in loneliness and depression.
4. Safety Concerns: Hearing is crucial for environmental awareness. People with untreated hearing loss may miss essential sounds like alarms, sirens, or approaching vehicles, which can put them or others at risk.

While some people believe they can manage their hearing loss without hearing aids, common coping strategies often fall short:

1. Lip Reading: While lip reading can help in some situations, it's not a foolproof method. Not all speech sounds are visible on the lips, and it can be challenging to rely on lip reading alone, especially in group settings or when the speaker is not facing you.
2. Increasing Volume: Turning up the volume on the TV or radio can help, but it's not a comprehensive solution. It doesn't improve clarity or the ability to distinguish between different sounds and can disturb others around you.
3. Avoidance: Many people with hearing loss avoid situations where they know they'll struggle to hear, such as social gatherings or noisy environments. This avoidance behavior can lead to further social isolation and emotional distress.

The myth that one can get by without hearing aids overlooks the significant impact of untreated hearing loss on communication, cognitive function, social engagement, and safety. While coping strategies may provide temporary relief, they do not address the underlying issue and can lead to further complications. Embracing hearing aids can significantly enhance the quality of life, offering clearer communication, cognitive benefits, social involvement, and increased safety.

Myth 5: I Don't Want to Admit That I Have Hearing Loss

Admitting to having hearing loss is a significant hurdle for many individuals. The reluctance often stems from various fears and misconceptions, including concerns about aging, stigma, and the perceived impact on one's lifestyle. However, acknowledging hearing loss is crucial for maintaining overall well-being and quality of life. Here's why the myth "I don't want to admit that I have hearing loss" is detrimental and why overcoming this denial is essential.

Before we can debunk the myth, we need to understand the reluctance.

1. Fear of Aging: One of the primary reasons people avoid admitting hearing loss is the association with aging. Hearing loss is often seen as a sign of getting older, which many people are reluctant to accept. This fear can lead to denial and a refusal to seek help.

2. Stigma and Self-Image: A stigma is attached to wearing hearing aids and acknowledging hearing loss. Many worry that admitting hearing loss will make them seem less capable or elderly. This concern about how others perceive them can prevent people from seeking the help they need.

3. Impact on Lifestyle: Some individuals believe that admitting to hearing loss will necessitate significant changes in their lifestyle. They may fear becoming dependent on hearing aids or believe their social and professional lives will suffer.

Now that we understand the reluctance, we can begin overcoming the myth with these truths.

1. Changing Perceptions: The first step in overcoming the reluctance to admit hearing loss is changing how it's perceived. Hearing loss should be seen as an ordinary and manageable condition, not as a sign of weakness or aging. Public awareness campaigns and education can help reduce the stigma associated with hearing loss and hearing aids.

2. Benefits of Early Detection: Acknowledging hearing loss early can lead to better outcomes. Early intervention can prevent further hearing deterioration, improve communication, and enhance overall quality of life. It's important to understand that hearing aids and other assistive devices can significantly improve life, not markers of decline.

3. Modern Hearing Aids: Technology advancements have made modern hearing aids much smaller, more effective, and more discreet than ever before. Many models are nearly invisible and offer features that can significantly improve hearing in various environments, making them a valuable asset rather than a burden.

4. Support Systems: Support from family, friends, and hearing health professionals can make a significant difference. Encouraging open conversations about hearing loss and seeking support can help individuals feel more comfortable admitting their condition and taking steps to address it.

The myth that "I don't want to admit that I have hearing loss" is a barrier that prevents many from seeking the help they need. Denial can lead to communication breakdowns, social isolation, cognitive decline, and safety risks. However, changing perceptions, understanding the benefits of early detection, embracing modern hearing aid technology, and seeking support can help individuals overcome this myth. Admitting hearing loss and taking proactive steps can improve communication, enhance quality of life, and improve overall well-being. If you suspect you have hearing loss, don't let denial hold you back—take the first step toward better hearing today.

Myth 6: Hearing Aids Will Make Everything Too Loud

A big misconception about hearing aids is that they will merely amplify all sounds, making everything louder rather than clearer. This misconception can lead to reluctance to seek help for hearing loss and prevent people from experiencing the significant benefits that modern hearing aids offer. In reality, contemporary hearing aids are sophisticated devices designed to enhance speech clarity and filter unwanted noise, thus improving the overall listening experience. Here's a closer look at why this myth is unfounded and how hearing aids work.

Many people hesitate to use hearing aids because they fear:

1. Overwhelming Noise: They believe hearing aids will amplify all sounds indiscriminately, making everyday environments overwhelming and uncomfortable.
2. Poor Sound Quality: There is a concern that hearing aids will not improve sound quality but will instead create a cacophony of loud noises.
3. Ineffectiveness: Some worry that hearing aids won't help them hear better in challenging listening situations, such as noisy restaurants or crowded places.

The reality is modern hearing aids are far more advanced than the rudimentary amplification devices of the past. Here's how they actually function:

1. Sound Processing and Customization

Today's hearing aids are equipped with digital signal processors that can distinguish between different types of sounds. These devices:

- Amplify Speech: They are specifically programmed to enhance speech frequencies, making conversations clearer.

- Reduce Background Noise: Advanced algorithms filter out background noise, such as traffic or crowd noise, allowing the wearer to focus on important sounds.

- Automatic Adjustments: Many hearing aids automatically adjust their settings based on the listening environment, ensuring optimal sound quality in various situations.

2. Directional Microphones

Modern hearing aids often feature directional microphones, which help focus on sounds coming from a particular direction (usually in front of the wearer) while reducing noise from other directions. This technology is particularly beneficial in noisy environments, as it helps the wearer concentrate on conversations without being overwhelmed by background noise.

To dispel the myth that hearing aids merely make everything louder, it's essential to:

1. Educate Yourself: Learn about the advanced technology used in modern hearing aids and how they can be customized to your hearing needs.
2. Consult a Professional: Visit an audiologist for a comprehensive hearing assessment and discuss your concerns. Audiologists can demonstrate how hearing aids work and

how they can be tailored to improve your hearing.
3. Trial Periods: Take advantage of trial periods offered by hearing aid providers. This allows you to experience the benefits of hearing aids in your daily life and make an informed decision.
4. Talk to Other Users: Hearing about the positive experiences of others who use hearing aids can provide reassurance and motivation to seek help for your hearing loss.

The myth that hearing aids will just make everything louder is rooted in outdated perceptions and a lack of understanding of modern hearing aid technology. Today's hearing aids are sophisticated devices designed to enhance speech clarity, reduce background noise, and provide a tailored listening experience. By addressing hearing loss with modern hearing aids, individuals can enjoy improved communication, enhanced quality of life, and better cognitive and overall health.

Myths of Addressing Hearing Loss

Myth 1: Hearing Aids Will Solve All My Communication Problems

The belief that hearing aids will solve all communication problems is a common misconception among those experiencing hearing loss. While modern hearing aids are highly advanced and can significantly improve hearing, they are not a magic bullet that resolves every communication challenge. Understanding the capabilities and limitations of hearing aids is essential for setting realistic expectations and achieving the best possible outcomes in managing hearing loss.

Modern hearing aids are sophisticated devices designed to enhance the auditory experience in numerous ways we've all explored. Despite these advanced features, hearing aids cannot resolve all communication issues. They can significantly improve hearing but do not restore it to normal levels or completely eliminate the challenges associated with hearing loss.

There are still limitations that a hearing aid wearer may face, including:

1. Environmental Noise: While hearing aids can reduce back-

ground noise, they cannot eliminate it entirely. In very noisy environments, even the best hearing aids may struggle to differentiate between speech and noise, leading to difficulties in understanding conversations.
2. Sound Localization: People with normal hearing can often determine the direction from which a sound is coming. This ability, known as sound localization, can be impaired in individuals with hearing loss, and hearing aids cannot fully restore this function.
3. Speech Understanding in Complex Situations: Hearing aids improve the audibility of speech but may not always enhance speech understanding, especially in complex acoustic environments where multiple people are talking at once.
4. Natural Sound Quality: Despite technological advances, hearing aids can sometimes produce a sound quality that is perceived as less natural compared to unaided hearing. Users might need time to adjust to these differences.

To address communication problems effectively, it is essential to complement hearing aids with other strategies and practices:

1. Communication Techniques: Effective communication is a two-way process. Both the person with hearing loss and their communication partners should be aware of techniques that facilitate better interactions. These include:
 - Face-to-face interaction: Ensuring the speaker faces the person with hearing loss can help with lip-reading and picking up visual cues.
 - Clear Speech: Speaking clearly, at a moderate pace, and not shouting can significantly improve understanding.
 - Rephrasing: If something is not understood, rephrasing the

sentence rather than just repeating it or saying it louder can help.

2. Captioning Services: Utilizing captioning services on TV shows, movies, and online videos or the phone can provide visual reinforcement to the auditory information, making it easier to follow along.

3. Environmental Modifications: Making changes to the environment can also aid communication. This can include reducing background noise by turning off the TV or radio during conversations, choosing quieter places for social interactions, and using soft furnishings to absorb sound and reduce echo.

4. Professional Support: Audiologists and hearing specialists can provide valuable support and advice on managing hearing loss. They can offer training in auditory rehabilitation, which focuses on improving listening skills and adapting to hearing aids.

Adjusting to hearing aids and managing hearing loss involves more than just the technical aspects. The psychological and emotional impact of hearing loss and the process of adapting to hearing aids should not be overlooked:

1. Acceptance and Realistic Expectations: Accepting that hearing aids will not solve all communication problems is crucial. Setting realistic expectations and being patient with the adjustment process can help mitigate frustration and disappointment.

2. Emotional Support: Hearing loss can lead to feelings of isolation and frustration. Seeking emotional support from friends, family, and support groups can provide comfort and understanding. Sharing experiences with others who have similar challenges can also be empowering.

3. Regular Follow-Ups: Regular follow-up appointments with an audiologist are essential to ensure that hearing aids are functioning optimally and to make any necessary adjustments. These appointments provide an opportunity to discuss any ongoing difficulties and explore additional strategies for improvement.

The myth that hearing aids will solve all communication problems is rooted in a misunderstanding of what these devices can and cannot do. While modern hearing aids offer significant benefits, they are not a cure-all for hearing loss. Understanding both your capabilities and limitations and the capabilities and limitations of your hearing loss is essential for setting realistic expectations and achieving the best possible outcomes.

Effective communication for individuals with hearing loss involves a multifaceted approach that includes hearing aids, complementary strategies, environmental modifications, and emotional support. By embracing a holistic approach to managing hearing loss, individuals can improve their communication, enhance their quality of life, and maintain their social and emotional well-being.

Recognizing that hearing aids are a valuable tool but not the sole solution is the first step toward successful hearing loss management. With the right combination of technology, strategies, and support, individuals with hearing loss can navigate their world more effectively and enjoy richer, more fulfilling interactions.

Myth 2: It's Too Late to Address My Hearing Loss

A myth that frequently comes up surrounding hearing loss is the belief that it's too late to address it. This misconception often leads individuals to forgo treatment, resigning themselves to a diminished quality of life. However, this belief is unfounded. It is never too late to seek help for hearing loss, and doing so can significantly improve one's quality of life, communication abilities, and overall well-being. Understanding the benefits of addressing hearing loss at any stage and debunking the myth of "too late" is essential for those living with this condition.

Hearing loss is a common issue that affects millions of people worldwide. According to the World Health Organization (WHO), around 430 million people globally have disabling hearing loss. In the United States alone, approximately 48 million people report some degree of hearing loss. While it is more prevalent among older adults, hearing loss can affect individuals of all ages. Despite its prevalence, many people delay seeking treatment due to misconceptions and fears, including the myth that it is too late to address their hearing loss.

Contrary to the myth, it is never too late to address hearing loss. Here are several reasons why seeking treatment at any stage can be beneficial:

1. Improved Communication: Hearing aids and other assistive devices can significantly enhance the ability to hear and understand speech, making communication more effective and enjoyable. This can lead to better relationships and a more active social life.
2. Cognitive Benefits: Treating hearing loss can help maintain cognitive function. Studies have shown that using

hearing aids can reduce the risk of cognitive decline and dementia. By providing the brain with the necessary auditory input, hearing aids help keep cognitive processes sharp.
3. Enhanced Quality of Life: Addressing hearing loss can substantially improve quality of life. Individuals seeking treatment often feel more confident, independent, and engaged in daily activities.
4. Increased Safety: Better hearing improves environmental awareness, allowing individuals to detect essential sounds that are crucial for safety. This can reduce the risk of accidents and enhance overall security.

Audiologists play a crucial role in the diagnosis and treatment of hearing loss. They can provide a comprehensive hearing assessment, recommend appropriate hearing aids or other assistive devices, and offer ongoing support and adjustments. Seeking the help of an audiologist can demystify the process and ensure that individuals receive the best possible care for their hearing needs.

In addition, hearing the experiences of others who have successfully addressed their hearing loss can be incredibly motivating. Many individuals report life-changing improvements after seeking treatment:

- Enhanced Relationships: Better hearing allows for more meaningful interactions with loved ones, improving relationships and social connections.
- Renewed Confidence: Hearing clearly boosts confidence in social and professional settings, leading to greater participation and engagement.
- Increased Independence: Improved hearing can make navi-

gating daily activities and environments easier.

The myth that it's too late to address hearing loss is not only false but also detrimental to those who believe it. Regardless of age or the duration of hearing loss, seeking treatment can significantly improve communication, cognitive health, social engagement, and overall quality of life. Modern hearing aids offer advanced technology that can be customized to individual needs, making them an effective solution for many people. Overcoming psychological barriers and seeking the help of audiologists can pave the way for a more fulfilling and connected life. It is never too late to take control of your hearing health and experience the benefits of better hearing.

Conclusion

By debunking these common myths and misconceptions, we hope to empower you to take control of your hearing health and explore the benefits of hearing aids. Remember, hearing loss is nothing to be ashamed of, and seeking treatment can improve your quality of life in countless ways. One thing that always comes up when people address their hearing concerns and start correcting their hearing is that it wasn't as hard or scary as they thought and that they wish they would've addressed it sooner!

Resources

- American Academy of Audiology Fact sheets: Hearing loss and depression (March 2018); Cognitive decline (January 2018); Age Related hearing loss (January 2018); Listening Effort and Fatigue (January 2018); Hearing loss (June 2017)
- Cool, Lisa Collier (2013). What do your ears reveal about your health? Healthy Hearing.
- Paker, Lisa (2015). Hearing Aids may help slow cognitive decline. Healthy Hearing.
- Signiausa (2016). Seniors are in denial about their hearing loss.
- Sturdivant, Grace Gore (2016). Cognitive Decline and Hearing Loss. Audiology Today. 16-21
- *Hearing loss statistics at a glance.* (2024, February 26). Healthy Hearing. https://www.healthyhearing.com/report/52814-Hearing-loss-statistics-at-a-glance#:~:text=According%20to%20the%20Centers%20for,at%20least%20some%20trouble%20hearing.
- World Health Organization: WHO. (2024, February 2). *Deafness and hearing loss.* https://www.who.int/news-room/fact-sheets/detail/deafness-and-hearing-loss
- *Research and tracking.* (2024, May 15). Hearing Loss in

Children. https://www.cdc.gov/hearing-loss-children/research/index.html#:~:text=CDC%20data%20have%20shown%20that,to%205%20per%201%2C000%20children.

About the Author

Daniel Troast is a licensed Doctor of Audiology with nearly 20 years of experience as an audiologist and hearing instrument specialist. He has a passion for educating individuals on the nuances of hearing loss and hearing aids. He has been interviewed by foxnews.com, thehealthy.com, cnet.com, and various other publications, as well as, been featured on several podcasts discussing hearing health.

www.ingramcontent.com/pod-product-compliance
Lightning Source LLC
Chambersburg PA
CBHW060616030426
42337CB00018B/3067